Living Longer

IS

the New Normal

Lessons from a Geropsychologist on Living Longer, Staying Positive, and Making it Over the Hurdles

Library of Congress Cataloging in Publication Data

Casciani, Joseph M.

Living Longer IS the New Normal

Library of Congress Control Number: 2020909873

ISBN: 9798649191210

Copyright © Living to 100 Club, LLC, 2020

Living to 100 Club SM and the tagline, Turning Aging on Its Head SM are protected, registered service marks with the U. S. Patent and Trademark Office.

All rights reserved.

No part of this book may be reproduced, stored in a retrieval system, or transmitted in any form or by any means, electronic, mechanical, photocopying, recording or otherwise, without the prior permission of the author.

First Edition

First Published 2020

To all of those elderly men and women in long-term care and in residential settings who have taught me so much about the human spirit, who have endured their medical and psychological conditions, and who have been brave and courageous in facing their setbacks, this book is respectfully dedicated.

CONTENTS

PREFACE 1

INTRODUCTION 4

SECTION 1: WHAT'S SO GREAT ABOUT AGING, ANYWAY?

Chapter 1: How Do I Start A New Chapter?...........................10

Chapter 2: What Color Is Your Setback?................................13

Chapter 3: How Do I Manage Setbacks?................................15

Chapter 4: What Can I Control?...19

Chapter 5: What Are the Strategies to Increased Longevity?... 22

Chapter 6: Where Can Determination Take Us?................... 26

SECTION 2: BODY, MIND, SPIRIT – STRATEGIES FOR HEALTHIER, LONGER LIVING

Chapter 7: Why Am I Not Defined By My Body?................... 30

Chapter 8: What Should I Know About Sexuality and Aging?... 32

Chapter 9: What Is Intermittent Fasting And Why Is It Important To Our Health?... 39

Chapter 10: What Educational Opportunities Are There For Seniors?... 46

Chapter 11: How One Exception Can Lift Our Depression 50

Chapter 12: What Do I Need To Know About Depression, Dementia and Delirium?... 53

Chapter 13: How Do I Individualize My Approach To Caregiving?.. 58

Chapter 14: Why Should I Be Good To Myself? 62

Chapter 15: Why Is Stepping Out Of My Comfort Zone So Important? 66

Chapter 16: What Does It Mean To Project A New Image On A Blank Screen? 68

Chapter 17: Why Does Worrying Get In the Way of Moving Forward? 72

SECTION 3: THE SCIENCE BEHIND AGING – AND BEING HAPPY ABOUT IT

Chapter 18: What Does Science Say About Living Longer Than We Think We Will? 76

Chapter 19: How Can I Better Understand Meaning and Purpose In Life? 80

Chapter 20: Age Is Only a Number 83

BIOGRAPHY 86

RECOMMENDED BOOKS AND RESOURCES 89

PREFACE

Just a little background. I am a psychologist with a specialty in geriatric mental health. Most of my work has been with older adults in nursing homes, where for over 30 years I have worked with individual patients, their families, and staff.

Then, I got the itch for more. I wanted to extend my reach beyond long-term care to individuals still living at home and who might want to know more about successful aging and longevity of life. But more than this – I am interested in how we adapt to setbacks and losses that inevitably come with aging. There is plenty of great information out there about how to improve diet, exercise, lifestyle habits, and other topics on the Internet, as well as in books and articles. But can knowing this information make us still stay positive after arthritis reduces our quality of life, when we can only get around with a walker, or if we have a leg that has been amputated?

Preface

I used to believe the mind and body cannot be separate. As a mental health professional, I used to think you can't treat the body without treating the psychological effects of the medical condition. We saw this all the time in nursing homes, where patients would be treated for, say, a breathing disorder, but who also needed help learning to cope with anxiety and panic – or the person with chronic pain who received physical therapy but needed a lot of help to deal with hopelessness. Then it became clearer we are not our body. They may be connected but when our body no longer cooperates we still have our mind, unless dementia appears but that's a conversation for another day. We always have the "me in there" that can have a positive outlook, the "me in there" that can still be determined to fight, and the "me" that can maintain motivation to get up every day and move forward.

This is the genesis of this book, **Living Longer IS the New Normal**, and the Living to 100 Club.

A note about article references:

Article references are noted in the book at the end of each chapter (where appropriate).

The format of the reference is as follows:

For print articles: Author name (year). Article title. *Publishing journal,* volume number (issue number), page range.

For online articles and websites: Author name (year). *Article or webpage title.* Publishing website. URL.

To gain access to these articles simply search for the article title in a search engine.

INTRODUCTION

Living Longer IS the New Normal is the creation of Dr. psychologist who has specialized in older adult care for over 30 years, including writing, public speaking, and providing training and support for scores of mental health professionals working in his professional corporations.

His experience in geropsychology has taught him many things:

- Age is only a number and does not say very much about what we should or should not be like.

- Older adults face many challenges, both normal and age-related changes, as well as unexpected problems and setbacks, both physical and mental.

- Proper medical care is essential, however, we also know our mental outlook – what we see in our future – has a huge impact on how well we manage these problems.

- How we interpret or explain life events can often color our ability to overcome them – or not. We face many challenges with advancing age – both age-related, like vision and hearing loss, and unexpected setbacks, like a stroke or broken hip – our mental outlook has a huge impact on how well we're going to manage these changes.

- We all have a vast reservoir of energy and creative spirit inside, sometimes untapped or blocked but it is always there. It explains how people can often accomplish things no one thought possible. When we can tap this internal energy, dig deep, and re-define ourselves as strong, resilient, and capable, we can take on a new challenge with a drive and determination we didn't know we had. Our reserve of motivation is bottomless – there is no end to what we can accomplish. And it is in every one of us.

This book is a frame of mind, a mindset, a metaphor for pushing ahead and maintaining a positive outlook about ourselves and our future. We are turning aging on its head! Living longer, happier, and healthier is an outcome of what we tell ourselves about our future and how we cope with stressful events. So, living to 100 is an important goal but it is more than a destination – it is the result of making the right choices and pushing forward. Whether we are still running marathons or confined to a wheelchair, living to 100 means staying positive in the face of change.

So, this book is the author's guide to creating and maintaining this positive frame of mind. The chapters in this book help readers examine usual thinking patterns about aging and encourage us to consider a different perspective on what we can accomplish and expect of ourselves. This is no time to sit back and muse "what will be will be" – it is time to re-define ourselves as strong and capable, and to shape our future as much as we can.

We also want to remember the future should be bigger than our past (see Dan Sullivan's website: www.strategiccoach.com).The point is not to dwell on our past or put our energies into longing for "the good old days" – they may provide great memories but if we get stuck in our past we don't move forward.

I speak in first person often throughout this book – as in what "I" as a Club Member believe, think, and feel. We can see this book as Club principles we hold as we face the future. If we take chronological age out of the equation and just set a goal to "live to 100" this is the outlook we aspire to. That is our goal. Join the **Club**, where Members are ***turning aging on its head***.

SECTION 1: WHAT'S SO GREAT ABOUT AGING, ANYWAY?

Chapter 1: How Do I Start A New Chapter?

Sometimes it's helpful to look back at our lives and see a series of chapters unfolding. These are not necessarily developmental stages, like childhood, young adulthood, and old age, but rather a succession of events or milestones that mark our journey, like graduation, marriage, birth of children, promotions, retirement, death of a spouse, and so on. These milestones serve as chapters in our life story.

With each new milestone, we must look at starting a new chapter, whether or not intended, pleasant or liberating. Situations like downsizing to a smaller home, divorce, getting rid of a car, having a stroke or heart attack, or experiencing the death of a spouse requires us to start a new chapter in our story. This is sometimes referred to as re-storying (refer to Gary Kenyon's work at the end of this book), where we look back at our life stories and ahead to our future and "write" new pages about how we have to take a new and different look at ourselves.

How can we go on after losing our spouse of 55 years? Many do not want to – it is just too painful, lonely, and dark facing the future alone. Of course, much time is needed to grieve and mourn this loss. Then we can decide to start a new chapter, continuing our odyssey now as a widow or widower, and start to redefine our self as someone who took an unexpected sharp turn and survived to live longer and stay positive – even in the face of challenge and loss.

We can recommend the same strategy to the husband or wife who is now a caregiver for their spouse who has debilitating Alzheimer's disease. It is time to write a new part for our self: *I'm now in the role of caring for my spouse, who needs my daily attention.* The point here is we are writing the script, taking on a new role in this next act, and creating whatever type of character we want to play.

This mindset also allows us to venture into new areas for work and leisure. Why not take classes in a new subject area – in person or online? And develop new skills, a new network of similar-minded individuals, and a new purpose. Ken Dychtwald, affiliated with his organization,

Age Wave (agewave.com), has written and researched this topic for decades and offers inspiration and insights on his website.

There is a wonderful movie produced by artist and photographer Lives Well Lived. Sky Bergman created this work to document many older adults who are thriving in their later years, many with challenges but who live successful, meaningful lives. It has been screened in many cities around the U.S. and is now available on her website www.lives-well-lived.com.

Living longer is about attitude, adapting, outlook, and staying positive – even when we experience adversity and setbacks.

Chapter 2: What Color Is Your Setback?

I'm aging every day. As I do, I face challenges that are both normal and age-related, as well as unexpected physical and mental setbacks. How I view my future has a major impact on how well I manage these challenges.

We can label this setback as just another sign of getting older or we can say, *Another bump in the road and I can get around this one, too.* There will always be bumps – no road is smooth all the way. If we interpret these as just part of the journey and see ourselves as capable and determined to move on then we will. On the other hand, if we say, *Oh, another setback, another surgery, another friend's death, another broken water pipe, I don't think I can handle another one,* that's when we lose our momentum and slow down and maybe pull off the road.

The best example here is probably the oldest: Is the glass half empty or half full? Person A says the stroke is something to adjust to and moves on and person B says it will change his life forever and nothing will be the same. They're both looking at the same event but each person is perceiving the outcome differently.

How we interpret or explain an event to ourselves will color how successfully we adapt to it.

Chapter 3: How Do I Manage Setbacks?

Successful confidence in aging involves maintaining as healthy a lifestyle as possible, watching our eating habits, staying physically active, having a sense of purpose, religious or spiritual ties, staying connected to family or a social group, and maintaining a positive mental attitude.

But what happens when a detour comes along on our successful aging journey? Maybe a stroke leaves us wheelchair-bound, a fall causes dislocated hip, we experience cognitive decline that impairs our ability to drive, or we get disabling arthritis – we all know diseases, complications, and accidents that can happen in old age is a long list.

Negative self-talk
Our self-talk is so important for our health and it plays a

huge role in how well we manage setbacks. When our inner dialogue is negative, it reinforces our self-limiting beliefs, adds stress, reduces our confidence and determination, and weakens our sense of control over the future. In short, it handicaps us.

In crude terms, carrying on this negative inner dialogue is like going into a butt-kicking contest with only one leg. The negative self-talk is a filter screening out good things and only allowing the bad to pass through. Once this thinking has taken over, we expect more of the same in the future. We extrapolate from this event that we are only in store for more. That inner voice just keeps repeating the words, *More of the same, My life is over, I'm ashamed to be in public, What kind of future do I have now, I don't have it in me to get through this*. And, most importantly, we close off that deep reservoir of energy we have inside. We reduce our inner flame to a single spark.

This energy fuels the drive and motivation that gets us back on the road. This flame ignites the belief that we are allowed to be happy – we *deserve* to be happy and the conviction this positive spirit is ours that no one can take away.

Successful Aging

Successful aging means choosing to be grateful for all

that has happened, even in the face of serious challenges. It means focusing on what we have and not on what we do not have. It means not comparing ourselves to others and certainly not basing our self-worth on accomplishments, failures, health, or sickness. Everyone has equal value and worth as a person, irrespective of whatever label or descriptor we assign. To age successfully underscores that everything is relative: there is always someone better off and someone who is worse off than I am.

The road ahead is not always smooth and well-paved. Accepting the cards we are dealt while fixing what we can and yet getting on with our lives means allowing the future to be bigger than our past. It means adapting to setbacks and moving on. It means solution-focused instead of emotion-focused coping. When we face a serious stress, we can either react emotionally and lose our effectiveness, or we can respond to the stress with a goal of finding solutions. And it means looking for new opportunities without the negative filters, regardless of our limitations. Maybe these words of the Dalai Lama will help us on this journey: *There are two days that we cannot get anything done – yesterday and tomorrow.*

It's important we recognize something that might make us want to give up and quit – loneliness, disease, death

– but in these setbacks we realize one important thing: we can *control our emotions* and get back to *healthy, happy living.*

Chapter 4: What Can I Control?

I understand I can't control most things but I can control my thoughts and feelings. How I interpret an event – a comment, a facial expression – impacts how I think and feel. As the Roman philosopher, Epictetus said, *We are disturbed not by events, but by the views we take of these events.* Negative thinking is associated with worrying, complaining, anger, blaming, and even feeling helpless. Positive thinking is associated with problem-solving, perseverance, planning, and possibility.

If we dig deep into this question of control, we can see there are many things we have no control over, like the weather or when the sun sets. Some things we do have partial control over, like our bank account balance or shooting 75 in a round of golf and some things we have complete control over, like our thoughts, values, and principles, and the goals we set for our self. It is pointless to fret over things we have no control over though perhaps we can and should take steps to reduce the impact of those things – steps like water conservation. Worrying about these things without taking preventive steps drains our energy and reduces our productivity. We can somewhat impact those we have some control over but what we should spend most of our time on is the third group – things we can fully control.

Even smiling, which is fully under our control, can lead to living longer. A study of professional baseball players who began their careers before 1950 found that after rating the intensity of player smiles in a sample of 230 photos those with bigger smiles lived an average of 7 years longer than those who were not smiling[1]. Though we should not assume that smiling contributes to living longer, we might infer from this study that whatever makes us choose to smile more may also contribute to accepting what we can and cannot control.

It is best to be aware of our thoughts, feelings, goals and principles – those things we can control – and not stress over what we have no say over. Pick our battles, as they say, and go after what we can shape and influence. There will always be negative, unpleasant events and knowing the difference leaves us with energy to win battles we can face and try to overcome. If you want to be part of the **Living to 100 Club** and stay around for a good long while, then you need to start looking at what situations and emotions are in your total control.

---

[1] Roan, S. (2010). *Life span may be as wide as your smile.* Los Angeles Times. latimes.com/archives/la-xpm-2010-mar-29-la-he-capsule-20100329-story

Chapter 5: What Are the Strategies to Increased Longevity?

Many large companies are always hunting for the next big breakthrough – the newest software or hardware that will change their systems, or the new operations that will keep them as cutting edge for their customers. The Chief Executive of Amazon, Jeff Bezos, however, has always taken the opposite position: what will not change in the next 10 years – what will be steady and predictable? The answer: to put it simply, what he and his top managers arrived at is that making things easy for customers will always be at the top of the customers' wish list. Everything revolves around this core principle at Amazon: provide the most convenience and the least friction possible for its customers, no matter what. That will not change.

Here at the Living to 100 Club, the focus is on successful aging, longevity, and managing setbacks. Our focus has one theme woven throughout articles, our radio show episodes, and other content. Whether the topic is on laughter, increasing exercise levels, or working beyond retirement age, the emphasis is always on coping with whatever struggle comes our way and facing the future with a positive mindset. On our live radio show, our guests contribute to this same perspective: sharing information that will help our audience take control of their future, take the right precautions, and manage setbacks, or learn to be better caregivers of others.

All of this brings me to the point of this chapter. New information about aging successfully and facing our advancing years with a positive outlook is all around us. But we already know what works. Here are the strategies, packaged a little differently:

- Everything is relative: if we only look for those who are healthier than us, we learn we can also find those who are sicker and more debilitated than we are. Or if they are wealthier or prettier, we can always find those who are less so. Be aware of comparisons and find the positive wherever we look.

- Be grateful for what we have. When it comes to

material possessions, Eric Hoffer had a memorable line, *You can never have enough of what you don't need to make you happy.* Focusing on what we do not have, disappointments or failures prevent us from seeing the whole picture as if we are wearing blinkers or blinders. With these on, we have no peripheral vision and all we see is what is directly in front of us: loss, disappointment, and everything that has gone wrong. Only when we remove the blinders can we see the whole picture – what is all around us – what we have as well as what we do not.

- Regular physical activity and movement are central ingredients to aging successfully. Research shows us time and again how exercise keeps us at our fittest. See the Appendix on recommended articles for more information.

- Take time for rest and relaxation, follow good stress reduction approaches like meditation, and get enough sleep.

- Remain connected to and engaged with family and friends. We should also think about expanding our circle of friends by associating with those who are younger than we are. Our closest group of life-long friends has a way of shrinking over time.

- Diet is central. Eat more whole-plant foods and less meat. Alcohol should be in moderation.

- Look for solutions but allow a measure of acceptance when there are none to be found. I like what Dr. Steven Gundry calls a *pessimistic optimism*: shrug our shoulders at the inevitable bad things that happen and celebrate the positives that do.

- Stay committed to a purpose – something that has meaning and brings a sense of enjoyment. Whether it is a religious or spiritual belief, connection to a community, or just a solo passion, hold on to something that is purposeful in our lives.

Of course, this list is but one perspective and there are many others. But, as we psychologists like to say, *process is more important than content*. Choosing to adopt any strategies is more important than the specific strategies we adopt.

Chapter 6: Where Can Determination Take Us?

I believe I have a vast reservoir of energy and creative spirit, sometimes untapped, and when I dig deep into this reservoir of energy, I can re-define myself as strong, resilient, and capable.

Each time we dig deep and accomplish something we did not think we were capable of doing our confidence builds and momentum keeps flowing. Sometimes we might be stunned by what we can achieve.

- *I never thought I could take 10 steps after my stroke, but I did.*

- *I never thought I could finish writing that chapter, it was the hardest one yet.*

- *I never thought I could make that phone call to my daughter after not talking for so long.*

- *I never thought I could give up my car keys – driving was always my lifeline – after getting lost too many times.*

- *I never thought I could talk with my neighbor again after what he said about my family.*

A single step is so hard, but we try and in trying we succeed. The best part is our success does not end. Whatever it took to take those extra steps, make that call, or change an opinion, we can find more of that determination and fire inside us so we can take on more battles. We are not going to experience just a single, major accomplishment but a succession of many more. The encouraging part about this is no one can take our drive and determination away from us – not our spouse, adult children, physician, or therapist. It is ours to keep forever.

SECTION 2: BODY, MIND, SPIRIT – STRATEGIES FOR HEALTHIER, LONGER LIVING

Chapter 7: Why Am I Not Defined By My Body?

I'd like to begin this section by first talking about the body. As we age, our physical appearance is among the first things we notice – small things like wrinkles around our eyes or a few gray hairs to bigger, more concerning things like muscle loss and skin loosening, illness, and disease. That is why these chapters are so important: so you can start seeing that *you are the captain of your ship*. Your body is the ship, and when you try to steer this body sometimes cooperates and sometimes it doesn't. As the captain, you have value and worth, regardless of your physical appearance or strength, or how sick or impaired your body is from chronic illness, stroke, amputation, or mental decline. *You are not defined by your body.*

I started calling one client *Captain* while helping her feel more in control and empowered after a stroke. I once asked her how her week was. She replied her ship ran aground and she fell while trying to walk. So, we turn the ship around and tried again.

It is quite easy to tie our value and worth to our well-being, our successes, or our health. This is a trap because our worth does not drop when we face failure or loss, or have a sharp physical decline. Our worth is intrinsic to being a living being. It is not based on what we can and cannot do, or what we have and do not have. It is the same trap children face when adults tie their worth and esteem to their academic achievements or work. Do we lose all self-esteem when we fail a class or get passed over for that promotion? Of course not.

When we understand that our worth and value as a person are not diminished by external or even internal events, we can remain forever positive about ourselves and we can empower others to believe it about themselves, too.

Captain your ship. Master the controls. And do not be afraid to try new, exhilarating things!

Chapter 8: What Should I Know About Sexuality and Aging?

There is an adage, *Older adults make love less often, but mean it more.* Sexuality in later life can remain constant and even though there may be some challenges, seniors can continue to enjoy a physically and emotionally fulfilling sex life at any age. As the adage implies, sex can be better at 70 or 80 and though it may not be what it was like at 20 or 30, fewer stresses and family and work demands, absence of unrealistic ideals and prejudices, less fear of unwanted pregnancy, and more privacy allows people to enjoy sex as much as or more than when they were younger.

The benefits of maintaining sexual activity[1] are well known, but some are less so:

- Sex burns fat and causes the brain to release endorphins, serving as natural pain killers and anxiety reducers.

- Sex prompts the release of substances that bolster the immune system and growth hormones, strengthening bones and muscles.

- Frequent sexual activity has been shown to slow the aging process and prevent wrinkles around the eyes.

- The physical exertion associated with sex is about the same as walking up two flights of stairs (and probably more pleasurable than what awaits you at the top!).

Some of the Common Things That Interfere with Sexual Activity

Science has taught us that normal aging brings physical changes for both men and women. An article from the National Institute on Aging[2] states changes for women are shortening and narrowing of the vagina, thinning of the vaginal walls, and less vaginal lubrication, making some types of vaginal activity painful or less desirable. For men, testosterone levels may decline and erectile dysfunction[3] (ED) becomes more common, interfering with how long it takes to get and maintain an erection or taking longer before another erection is possible.

Other barriers that accompany the normal aging process include changes in body image with new questions about how "attractive" we are to our partner, performance anxiety and worry about sexual attention[4], major lifestyle changes such as retirement, and new concerns about illness, physical problems and surgeries. Finally, we are never too old to worry about the risk of sexually transmitted diseases when engaging in sexual activity with another person who has other sexual partners – old age does not protect us from diseases like genital herpes, hepatitis B, or HIV.

Physical and Psychological Changes Impacting Sexual Activity

Many illnesses, disabilities, and medications can impact the older adult's sex life. These include:

- Diabetes – frequently causes ED in men or vaginal yeast infections in women.

- Chronic pain – interferes with physical intimacy, while pain medication itself can interfere with sexual function.

- Heart disease – interferes with circulation, complicating physical arousal.

- Heart attack – not necessarily interfering with the

enjoyment of an active sex life, a history of heart attack can increase fear of sexual activity triggering another – though these fears are generally unfounded.

- Dementia – affects judgement, appropriateness, and even recognizing his or her partner.

- Incontinence – results in loss of bladder control during sex.

- Stroke – often causes weakness or paralysis in different parts of the body.

- Surgery (e.g. hysterectomy, mastectomy, or prostatectomy) – creates worry about future sex, loss of interest, or feeling less desirable.

- Medications – many prescription drugs used to treat high blood pressure, cancer, ulcers, anxiety, and depression have side effects that impact sexual function and sexual desire.

- Smoking and excess alcohol – though strictly lifestyle choices, both have a deleterious effect on sexual function.

Know When to Seek Help

Check with your physician or mental health professional

about:

- Switching medications with fewer side effects if your drug treatment limits your sexual enjoyment or functioning.

- Cardiac rehabilitation programs to improve physical fitness.

- Fear and worry about losing sexual interest and desire, low self-esteem, how attractive we are, or difficulty coping with new life stresses – whether or not these are age-related.

- Erectile dysfunction or vaginal discomfort and seeking the treatments that are readily available.

Adapting – What It's All About!

Every physical and psychological change that comes with advancing age requires new approaches to maximize our enjoyment of sexual activity. Bodily changes in weight, skin and muscle tone require us to look beyond our own physical appearance and that of our partners, to feel just as comfortable in our aging body as we did in our young body, and to not let blame or judgement get in the way of enjoying a fulfilling sex life.

Feel free to be open with your partner about your sexual

expectations and anxieties. Discover new ways to be physically intimate if there are new obstacles. If sexual intercourse is not possible, look for new ways to restore emotional and physical intimacy to a relationship.

Be willing to take more time to set the stage for romance and intimacy. If you have lost your partner due to severe physical impairment or death, or through separation or divorce, start a new chapter and imagine beginning another relationship, and consider exploring social dating sites[5]. No one outgrows the need for intimacy and emotional closeness. If we are joining the Living to 100 Club, *amore* must be in the picture!

---

[1] Public Health Agency of Canada. (September 2006). *Seniors and Aging - Sexual Activity*.
publications.gc.ca/collections/collection_2007/hc-sc/H13-7-15-2006E.pdf

[2] National Institute on Aging. (2017). *Sexuality in Later Life*.
nia.nih.gov/health/sexuality-later-life

[3] For a current list of must-read books about erectile dysfunction visit edtreatment.info

[4] Segal, M. & Smith, M. (2019). *Better Sex as You Age*. HelpGuide.
helpguide.org/articles/alzheimers-dementia-aging/better-sex-as-you-age.htm

[5] For a list review of the best senior dating sites go to retirementliving.com/best-senior-dating-sites

Chapter 9: What Is Intermittent Fasting And Why Is It Important To Our Health?

A subject I have become interested in recently is intermittent fasting (shortened to "IF" for this chapter). This has become a trend for the health-conscious population as a way to not only lose weight but also, according to many research studies, reduce disease and slow down the aging process. It basically refers to eating patterns that cycle between periods of fasting and eating – eating within a specific timeframe and fasting for the rest of the time. It is typically seen as more of a lifestyle choice than a diet.

Intermittent fasting is nothing new. Throughout evolution, our ancestors often fasted because food was not always available and the hunting and foraging process often left people cycling between the time of food abundance and scarcity. Further, Christian, Jewish, and Buddhist traditions, among others, have frequently included fasting as part of their religious practice.

Variations

IF comes in many variations:

- 5:2 method – normal eating five days a week and reduced calorie intake (500 to 600 calories) the other two days.

- Eat-stop-eat – restricted eating for 24 hours once or twice a week.

- 16/8 – consume any desired calories within a 6- to 8-hour period and fasting the remaining 14 to 16 hours.

- Any similar combinations or permutations marked with periods (hours or days) of reduced calorie intake.

Favorable Outcomes

There is no shortage of articles and research findings on the practice of IF. Among the many benefits touted include weight loss, increased energy, cellular repair, and other highly desirable effects. Many of these studies involved small sample sizes or were limited to animal studies so there are still many questions yet to be answered with the effects on humans. The research is promising, nonetheless:

- Improved insulin sensitivity and lowered insulin levels, which makes stored body fat more accessible[1]

- Benefits of fat loss and muscle gain due to up to five times increase in human growth hormone[2]

- Changes in gene function, related to longevity and the protection from disease[3;4]

- Boosts metabolism and increases the release of fat-burning norepinephrine, which is directly related to weight loss[5;6]

- Reducing inflammation, precursors to many chronic diseases[7]

- Protection against neurodegenerative disorders[8], coronary artery disease[9], metabolic disturbances[10], and diabetes[11].

Although there is abundant research (as the above citations show) reporting how intermittent fasting slows aging, a recent study at Harvard[12] explored *the underlying biology* of the way our cells process energy over time – a process associated with aging and age-related disease. The subjects were earthworms and the study looked at molecules contained in the cell's mitochondria and how well these mitochondria provided cells with sources of energy throughout the worm's (short) life. When diets were restricted these mitochondrial networks were kept in a "youthful" state. The authors confirmed that low-energy conditions, such as dietary restriction, do promote healthy aging, but they also show the biological processes occurring with these dietary restrictions.

Contraindications

There are some risks from IF with people who are underweight or have a history of eating disorders and has also been shown to have undesired effects on menstrual cycles and fertility[13] in some women. Other contraindications are those with diabetes, problems regulating sugar levels, or when taking certain medications. It is advisable to consult with your physician before deciding to partake in an IF program.

IF can have many benefits for our body and brain, including living longer. The diet tends to help us take in fewer calories while burning more calories. Although there are many favorable outcomes, I think it is important to remember that IF represents a lifestyle change. The process has been beneficial for me, initially abstaining from food for 24 hours a week (actually 36, but we do not eat while sleeping) for about 8 months, and gradually adding in dinner on the day of fasting. My total weight loss to date has been about 30 pounds. It is not for everybody, but once risks have been ruled out, I highly recommend it.

---

[1] Heilbronn, L.K., Smith, S.R., Martin, C.K., Anton, S.D. & Ravussin, E. (2005). Alternate-day fasting in nonobese subjects: effects on body weight, body composition, and energy metabolism. *Am J Clin Nutr*. 81(1), 69-73.

[2] Ho, K. Y., Veldhuis, J. D., Johnson, M. L., Furlanetto, R., Evans, W. S., Alberti, K. G. & Thorner, M. O. (1988). Fasting enhances growth hormone secretion and amplifies the complex rhythms of growth hormone secretion in man. *The Journal of clinical investigation*, 81(4), 968-975.

[3] Martin, B., Mattson, M. P. & Maudsley, S. (2006). Caloric restriction and intermittent fasting: two potential diets for successful brain aging. *Ageing research reviews*, 5(3), 332-353.

[4] Goodrick, C. L., Ingram, D. K., Reynolds, M. A., Freeman, J. R. & Cider, N. L. (1982). Effects of Intermittent Feeding Upon Growth and Life Span in Rats. *Gerontology*, 28, 233-241.

[5] Gunners, K. (2017). *How Intermittent Fasting Can Help You Lose Weight*. Heathline. www.healthline.com/nutrition/intermittent-fasting-and-weight-loss

[6] Barnosky, A. R., Hoddy, K. K., Unterman, T. G. & Varady, K. A. (2014). Intermittent fasting vs daily calorie restriction for type 2 diabetes prevention: a review of human findings. *Translational Research*, 164(4), 302-311.

[7] Johnson, J. B., Summer, W., Cutler, R. G., Martin, B., Hyun, D. H., Dixit, V. D., Pearson, M., Nassar, M., Telljohann, R., Maudsley, S., Carlson, O., John, S., Laub, D. R. & Mattson, M. P. (2007). Alternate day calorie restriction improves clinical findings and reduces markers of oxidative stress and inflammation in overweight adults with moderate asthma. *Free radical biology & medicine*, 42(5), 665-674.

[8] Lee, J., Duan, W., Long, J. M., Ingram, D. K. & Mattson, M. P. (2000). Dietary restriction increases the number of newly generated neural cells, and induces BDNF expression, in the dentate gyrus of rats. *Journal of molecular neuroscience*, 15(2), 99-108.

[9] Varady, K. A., Bhutani, S., Church, E. C. & Klempel, M. C. (2009). Short-term modified alternate-day fasting: a novel dietary strategy for weight loss and cardioprotection in obese adults. *The American journal of clinical nutrition*, 90(5), 1138-1143.

[10] Reis de Azevedo, F., Ikeoka, D. & Caramelli, B. (2013). Effects of intermittent fasting on metabolism in men. *Revista da Associação Médica Brasileira*, 59(2), 167-173.

[11] Also see Barnosky, A. R., Hoddy, K. K., Unterman, T. G. & Varady, K. A. (2014).

[12] Harvard Chan School. (2017). *In Pursuit of Healthy Aging*. The Harvard Gazette. news.harvard.edu/gazette/story/2017/11/intermittent-fasting-may-be-center-of-increasing-lifespan

[13] Martin, B., Pearson, M., Brenneman, R., Golden, E., Wood, W., Prabhu, V., Becker, K. G., Mattson, M. P., & Maudsley, S. (2009).

Gonadal transcriptome alterations in response to dietary energy intake: sensing the reproductive environment. *PloS one*, 4(1).

Chapter 10: What Educational Opportunities Are There For Seniors?

We do not just need to think about our bodies – sexually or through healthy eating – we also need to be more conscious of nurturing our mind. Keeping an active mind is known to help cognitive function, reduces stress, and combined with the right diet and exercise, can contribute to a longer life.

Years ago, a young gerontologist/psychologist by the name of Ken Dychtwald, PhD (visit agewave.com for information about Ken) shared his vision for the aging socicty based on the changing demographics occurring in the United States. He saw how changes in longevity, interests, and lifestyle would create a shift in our thinking about "growing old" and how the traditional, linear, and predictable retirement process would become cyclic, with opportunities for second and third careers, new social networks, and deep changes in our thinking about what we are capable of with advancing age. Dr. Dychtwald has since become the foremost thinker and visionary regarding the marketing, health care, and workforce implications of the burgeoning older adult population. His company, Age Wave, guides companies and government groups in product and service development for older generations.

Today, retirees and pre-retirees are seeking new vocations, volunteer opportunities, and paid positions that are either in line with their careers or completely different from their life-long work history. This chapter offers some of the leading sites for adult online learning, covering virtually any topic where you can work at your own pace from your own home or office, and learn new skills needed to pursue your goals. Many sites offer free courses – some have partnered with leading universities, some offer credit toward undergraduate and graduate degrees, and some just provide "lessons worth sharing" for the curious adult learner.

Here are some of the best websites for adult online learning:

Carnegie Mellon University Open Learning Initiative (oli.cmu.edu/independent-learner-courses) – course materials available at no charge, focusing on high-quality, scientifically based lessons.

Coursera (techboomers.com/t/what-is-coursera) – university-based online courses matching the same classes that are taught at various accredited universities around the world.

edX (edx.org) – an extensive list of global educational partners with MOOC (massive open online courses), many offering certificates and credits that can be applied toward college degrees.

GCF Learn Free (edu.gcfglobal.org) – tutorials on using the digital world and for beginners who are new to using computers, including smartphones and tablets, social media, and computer basics.

LearnMyWay (learnmyway.com) – onsite learning opportunities for those who want to learn to use the Internet, with topics on emails, online shopping, safety and privacy, and public services online.

Lynda (lynda.com) – now named LinkedIn Learning, this is an educational website with over 4,500 courses on business, creativity, and technology-related topics, though this is a subscription-based website.

OpenEdu (open.ac.uk) – based in the United Kingdom,

this site is touted as an open university: open to people, places, ideas, and methods.

Open Yale Courses (oyc.yale.edu) – operated by Yale University, an extensive catalog of online courses that can be searched and filtered by discipline and field.

TechBoomers (techboomers.com) – oriented toward general internet and technology knowledge, learn how to use popular websites and apps and "improve your life with technology".

TED Ed (ed.ted.com) – a site supporting learning in general, with access to text lessons, videos, and interactive lessons on over 200,000 topics.

Udemy (udemy.com) – choose from a library of over 45,000 courses. Includes extensive course details about how long each course will take, as well as lectures and videos, required skill level, and other information.

So, there is no shortage of opportunities to change our thinking about growing old and instead to shift into a mode of acquiring new skills and talents and pursue interests that may have long been put on hold. And again, process is more important that content: the mere act of doing trumps what we actually do.

Chapter 11: How One Exception Can Lift Our Depression

Depression affects us in many ways and one thing it does well is narrow our perspective. When someone is depressed, all they see are the wrongs, failures, disappointments, and everything that has not gone as desired. Depression blocks our vision and limits us from seeing the whole picture. It acts as a filter, only letting in the bad and keeping out the good.

To remove the filter, we need to find exceptions, even a single exception that something – one thing – has gone right. *The food tastes terrible here, my children never seem to care, I am just worthless to everyone – there is nothing good about being alive.* Can you find one exception – maybe the one person who is different from the rest, one meal you do look forward to, one bright spot about your family, or one small sign that someone really does care?

Once you notice the exception you can build on it. Just as someone who only sees her physical decline, arthritis, vision and hearing problems, difficulty sleeping, we have to look for strengths (referred to as "residual strengths"), those things that are still intact and what we are still good at. Exceptions are always there – sometimes they are hard to see but they are there.

Exceptions can lead the way to changing our perceptions and removing the negative filters so we see a more complete picture.

As highlighted in previous chapters, focusing only on what we don't have and our disappointments or failures limits our peripheral vision where all we see is what's directly in front of us: everything that's gone wrong. There comes a time when we need to remove the blinkers so we can see the whole picture – what is all around us – the right and not just the wrong.

Often, depression can also seem like a vacuum, pulling us back into a void – a deep hole of darkness – and no matter how hard we try to pull away, we fall back into the same hole. Of course, there are other, perhaps more clinical ways to describe the process of becoming depressed, but this visualization helps many people. Forcing ourselves to not yield to this dark place and resisting the pull backward is the way we can overcome it. Resisting that pull, seeking the positives that lie ahead, and setting a goal that pushes us forward can make all the difference. Even when the temptation to retreat to this dark place is so strong and can even seem so comforting and safe, it must be resisted. Yielding to this pull backward only makes the hole deeper and makes it more difficult for us to recover from. A Christine Caine quote conceptualizes a nice shift in our perspective, *Sometimes when you're in a dark place, you think you've been buried, but actually you've been planted.*

Look for the exception, the solution, the shift in perception to fight this backward pull. Just like when we only seeing dark clouds when we are depressed, we can understand there is always a blue sky above the clouds. Allowing a little blue to poke through the gray skies is your exception. Eventually, depression's dark clouds start to dissipate and we can see a little more of the blue sky than we did before.

Chapter 12: What Do I Need To Know About Depression, Dementia and Delirium?

This chapter is about three clinical syndromes that besiege many older adults: depression, dementia, and delirium. For those who may have heard these terms but do not know how to distinguish one from the other, this chapter sets out to provide you with a little more knowledge about similarities and differences.

Why is this an important subject? Caregivers – both paid and unpaid – make up 20% of the U.S. population and this is expected to grow rapidly over the coming decades for several reasons: demographics, an aging population, medical advances that allow for shorter hospital stays, and better technology that allows people to stay in their homes for longer. Additionally, at least 30% of caregivers are caring for someone with cognitive impairment (according to caregiver.org).

Depression, dementia, and delirium are colloquially referred to as the "3 D's".

First, what does **depression** look like?

- Sad mood, feeling worthless, hopeless, and helpless
- Loss of interest in activities, decreased energy, and loss of initiative
- Feelings of guilt and remorse, preoccupations with disappointment and failure
- Disruptions in sleep and eating habits
- Difficulty with attention and concentration

In addition to these signs, we need to watch for increased isolation and withdrawal, persistent complaints of memory problems, somatic complaints – usually vague and hard to assess – self-neglect, aimless and purposeless attitudes, and expressions of disinterest in living life.

Thoughts of self-harm, including suicide, sometimes occur for depressed individuals, especially when we see non-compliance with medical plans, reckless behavior, misuse of alcohol or other drugs, or expressions of feeling trapped or unable to improve the situation.

Dementia is a global or diffuse change in our mental or cognitive abilities. Dementia is typically irreversible (when caused by certain diseases like Alzheimer's, Parkinson's, vascular changes, and infections or severe trauma). Though rare, some dementing conditions are reversible if caused by nutritional deficiencies, over-medication, and severe environmental stress. These latter conditions can reverse when the individual has proper medical workup and treatment. Even depression can mimic the signs of dementia due to cognitive complaints, listlessness, and loss of initiative – all common in both conditions. The cognitive changes we see in dementia include memory loss – usually short-term memory – loss of factual information, difficulty with attention and concentration, emotional lability and reduced frustration tolerance, gradual disorientation, and most commonly, difficulty with word-finding and self-expression.

Distinguishing between the two conditions is not a simple matter, as both depression and dementia have similar features. However, depression tends to have a more sudden onset, whereas dementia is a slow, insidious process. Waking early is more common in depression than in dementia. Most importantly, there is a greater incidence of self-reported or exaggerated loss in depression. In contrast, individuals with dementia tend to mask or downplay their losses. Sundowning, marked by increased confusion and disorientation later in the day and early evening, is common in dementia. Lastly, depression tends to be marked with difficulty with recent *and* remote memory function, while remote memory in individuals with dementia tends to be better preserved.

The third "D" is **delirium**, characterized by a rapid onset and global cognitive impairment. Signs of delirium include a disturbance in consciousness (sometimes referred to as "acute confusional state"), perceptual disturbances, disturbed sleep-wake cycle, disorganized thinking, altered attention levels and high distractibility. The important feature about delirium is that it is a medical emergency and the cause needs to be identified urgently. Causes include stroke, infection, adverse drug reactions, and post-anesthesia or post-operative conditions.

Highlighting the differences between dementia and delirium would focus on:

- Onset – sudden with delirium and slow with dementia
- A normal state of consciousness with dementia and fluctuating consciousness with delirium
- Perceptual disturbances (hearing a door slam and

thinking it is a gunshot) is present in delirium but not in dementia

- A disturbed sleep-wake cycle and high levels of distractibility occur in delirium but not in dementia.

A chapter of a book is limited space in which to give this subject its due. But, pushing forward to live as successfully as possible in our later years and as caregivers for our relatives and close friends means we must be informed. Having facts at our disposal to make important, necessary health care decisions, and to bring concerns to health professionals is imperative in depression, dementia, and delirium support.

Chapter 13: How Do I Individualize My Approach To Caregiving?

Living longer means physical decline is more likely to accompany our later years, whether in our sensory systems, agility, balance, mental function, communication skills, or the myriad chronic diseases we see in old age. And, as our population ages, more caregiving is being provided by family members and other caregivers who are not paid health care professionals. A report by the Mayo Clinic[1] found around 1 in 3 adults in the US provides care to other adults as informal caregivers.

There are many recommended strategies for caregivers to reduce their level of stress and burnout – accepting help, joining a support group, staying connected with others, and other useful steps. One approach often overlooked is the notion of prevention, accomplished by individualizing the way we interact with the family member who needs some level of care.

Caregiving comes in all shapes and sizes, depending on the functional capacities of the care recipient. Whether the caregiver is a spouse, sibling, or parent, we know that caring for a frail, bed-ridden person requires strategies that differ from those needed for a different person, such as one with moderate to advanced dementia living at home. Nonetheless, underlying all care at home – and in any setting – is understanding the elements of two-way communication and tolerance for uniqueness. This means individualizing our approach to the unique needs of the care recipient, focusing on listening more than advising, and collaborating on solutions. These approaches will be more effective in the long run and more respectful of the person we are helping.

Individualized Care Means Two-way Communication

Our loved ones must have an opportunity to ask questions, voice their anxieties and fears about what can be expected in their future, and have a say in what goals should be set in their care. One-way communication from the caregiver to the care recipient is an outmoded approach and is not effective for providing the help a care recipient needs to adapt successfully to the changes he or she is facing. We increase the chances of better coping when the care recipient has enough information to make informed decisions and becomes part of the long-term goals for their life and future. When we overlook or minimize the person's involvement in their own care and we do not take the time to really hear what they want, compliance is likely to be superficial and temporary and often creates a decline in functioning.

Individualized Care Means Understanding the Diverse Interests and Needs of Our Loved Ones

Acknowledging that a parent or spouse will voice different needs than what we believe are right is conducive to complying with the overall care plan. That is, the caregiver may not agree with the expressed desires of this parent or spouse but understanding these desires and finding some way to accommodate them is an important ingredient of being a successful caregiver. Allowing mom to visit friends or continue her weekly swimming classes creates opportunities for maintaining her quality of life and also respects the person's remaining decision-making capacity. Or signing up the husband with Alzheimer's disease for harmonica lessons – an activity that is very plausible for certain dementias – offers relief and gratification for the caregiver. True, we must manage the risks that come with this level of independence, but we also know that compromises and alternative solutions are always available. We want to protect a family member from possible harm, but allowing the person to stay involved in activities of daily living or self-care fosters a sense of purpose, meaning, and keeps the fire burning.

---

[1] Mayo clinic staff. (2020). *Caregiver stress: Tips for taking care of yourself.* Mayoclinic. www.mayoclinic.org/healthy-lifestyle/stress-management/in-depth/caregiver-stress/art-20044784

Chapter 14: Why Should I Be Good To Myself?

A newspaper article highlighted the important notion of self-care: be good to yourself first – others come later. The article was written about a Buddhist monk Haemin Sunim, who has just published his latest book, *Love for Imperfect Things*. Sunim is a popular Buddhist teacher and spiritual guide, espousing the subjects of managing stress and overcoming the challenges of everyday life, especially through the power of self-care. He says we should not forget we have a responsibility to be good to our self before anything else.

In the Living to 100 Club, we talk a lot about healthy lifestyles, the road to living longer, and how to manage setbacks that inevitably occur with age. In one of our recent live radio shows on Voice America, *Better Habits, Better Health,* we talked with Dr. Michael Howard, a health educator. He summarized those lifestyle steps that contribute to the longest, happiest, and healthiest lives: maintaining our weight, adding more plant-based foods to our diet, regular exercise, no smoking, and alcohol in moderation.

Haemin Sunim, however, adds five elements of self-care to this list that involves taking time for our self to focus on our own needs, and cautions us to do so without feeling selfish:

- **Breathe** – start by taking a deep breath, being mindful of our breathing, and observe how it becomes deeper the more we focus on it, which in turn helps us feel more centered and calmer. Just focusing and paying attention to it a few minutes a day helps us to become more mindful and centered.

- **Accept** – our self and our many imperfections. As Sunim says, *The path to self-care starts with acceptance, especially of our struggles.* When we accept these struggles and stop trying to overcome them, the mind stops struggling and grows quiet. Trying to change or control difficult emotions works against our self-care, as does striving for perfection.

- **Write** – put pen to paper those things weighing on us and the things we need to do while unloading them from our head and heart. Once on paper and after a night's rest, whatever steps we need to take are more obvious and more manageable.

- **Talk** – As any psychologist will tell you, speaking with a non-judgmental friend or relative about our frustrations or difficult feelings will lighten the burden we carry. But, more importantly, the answers we already had inside are now more obvious when talking with another person and are more objective.

- **Walk** – Just walking helps to distract the mind and *create space between the mind and whatever is causing distress.* Instead of sitting and dwelling on what is burdening us, the changes in our physical energy that come from walking allow us to get out of our head and observe what is around us, thereby releasing the stresses within. This step certainly fits with another book by Sunim, *The Things You Can See Only When You Slow Down.*

We consider it important to be good to others, but it is beneficial we do not forget to be kind to ourselves in the process. Sometimes being good to ourselves means changing our habits so we can lead happier and more fulfilling lives.

Chapter 15: Why Is Stepping Out Of My Comfort Zone So Important?

Being unpredictable adds excitement. I like to occasionally step out of my comfort zone – in what I say, what I do, and even what I wear – because it triggers different reactions from family, co-workers, and friends, and opens a world of new social interactions and opportunity. As we know, our comfort zone is that familiar, comfortable place where we feel safe and secure, and where we act and speak consistently and predictably. Stepping out of that comfort zone triggers comments, like *Why is he acting so strange – is he on something?* Or *That was an unusual thing for you to say.* We like to be predictable because it invites calmness and dispels anxiety. Why unnecessarily create uneasiness?

In his book, *Breaking the Habit of Being Yourself*, Dr. Joe

Dispenza explains how shifting away from our usual behavior patterns into unknown territory creates new and exciting opportunities in our life odyssey. As we develop new relationships, enjoy new experiences and elicit different reactions from those closest to us, more opportunity awaits and more doors open. Do we take drum lessons when we never had any musical interest before? Do we go out to dinner with neighbors we barely know? Do we volunteer to do something we have never had an interest in?

Predictability and routine life are safe. Stepping out of our comfort zone, however, keeps us alert and open to new possibilities, which in turn provide endless sources of energy, drive, and spirit.

So, try something new and stay out of your comfort zone – be the unpredictable while we explore all our inner dimensions. You never know what new passions you might find.

Chapter 16: What Does It Mean To Project A New Image On A Blank Screen?

There is beauty in being open to a new, positive future. I can create a new definition of myself as I want it to be – I am not stuck with how I defined myself yesterday. Like any construction, we can remodel our self-definition because as we mentally define ourselves we can just as easily redefine.

Steve Jobs, the creator of Apple, was given up for adoption by his birth parents. When he found out about this at a young age he felt totally worthless. He felt sure he would never accomplish anything because he was unwanted by his biological mother and father. Jobs was experiencing negative self-talk: *I am not worthy of others; I am empty and unlovable.* But his adoptive parents explained he was the most beautiful and smartest person in the world, even as a child, and that was why they adopted him. This was positive self-talk: *maybe I am lovable and capable and maybe I have some value as a person after all.*

After that conversation with his adoptive parents, Steve Jobs re-defined himself. The definition was new, but the young adult who once had such a negative self-image now had turned this image into a positive one. He had not changed – there were no new skills or talents bestowed on him by the couple who adopted him. It was like flipping a light switch and his self-perception went from dark to light. It was simply his mental construction of himself that changed – the self-talk going on in his head.

Our self-talk can be pessimistic, like Steve Jobs before the heart-to-heart with his parents, or as aspirational as his self-talk became after this talk. We are not defined by who we were or what we believed in the past. Instead, we can create our own self-definition, re-shape our identity and sharpen our ability to face daily challenges. If we are discouraged by failure and disappointment in the past, we do not have to be discouraged again in the months and years ahead. Do not let yesterday define who you are today. Remember – there is always a blank screen in front of us.

Another perspective on digging deep and finding new dimensions to our sense of self we never saw before is found in the famous Renaissance architect, painter, and sculptor Michelangelo Buonarroti, who was highly esteemed for his statues, created from blocks of marble and granite. He has been described as one of the greatest artists of all time. He sculpted two of his best-known works, the Pieta and the statue David before the age of 30. Born in 1475 and dying in 1564 at the age of 88, he was still admired for his *terribilita* – what his contemporaries referred to as his ability to instill a sense of awe in his works.

Many of Michelangelo's quotes are memorable. Two that stand out are attributed to his work. Michelangelo was once asked how he could create such breathtaking, beautiful works of art from a block of stone. His reply: *Every block of stone has a statue inside it, and it is the task of the sculptor to discover it.* And another quote, he says, in an affirmation of his *terribilita*, *I saw the angel in the marble and carved until I set him free.*

So much goes on in our head that we can create negative self-talk patterns that greatly influence how we face the future or even our perception of reality in the moment. We have a blank screen to project our new image, or a new block of marble to create a new identity, adding all the features, attitudes, and character that we want. Why not let the positive spirit, optimism, and energy create the lines of this new self-image? Why not let positive self-talk take over this time?

Chapter 17: Why Does Worrying Get In the Way of Moving Forward?

It is difficult to change your internal chatter to positive self-talk when we have the burden of worry to carry.

Worry is unpleasant but it can also be soothing and comforting, much like a good, familiar friend. We like to keep it around. Some believe it helps to cope with problems and for us to prepare for the worst. But worry is also described as *borrowing trouble from the future*. It usually starts with questions about the future, *What if ... happens?* And reflects our uneasiness about being unable to predict the future. Much like our comfort zone, we like predictability.

Sometimes, worry is related to an inability to tolerate uncertainty. Ambiguity is stressful and is viewed as a threat by some people: *I can't live with not knowing, so*

I'm going to predict the worst and just dwell on this. Even though the imagined threat increases our anxiety, it is something to hold on to and become preoccupied with, like a security blanket we had as children. *I've had a series of mini-strokes: I know I'll have another; I might as well accept it and get prepared for it.* Awfulizing is another way to describe this pattern: *My future looks awful; everything I see is awful.*

We do not know for sure what is going to happen and when we spend time imagining the worst and predicting calamity or catastrophe, this mindset generally results in reduced quality of life. Despite how soothing it can be, we know worrying helps no one, it drains energy – stopping us from being more productive – and it interferes with planning our tomorrows. It also interferes with problem-solving and decision-making, so in worrying about our future we make poor choices, outcomes of which lead to more worrying. In the end, this type of thinking is cyclical and it can be very difficult to stop. Worrying is akin to our negative self-talk we spoke about in the previous chapter: unhelpful thoughts such as, *What's the use? I know I'm going to lose my vision anyway.*

We need to accept a certain amount of uncertainty and ambiguity in our lives. Explore the works of those who believe in the Law of Attraction[1] and one of its tenets:

What we think about, we bring about. Research the many books and articles on how to reduce worry[2]. One common element in these approaches is recognizing the importance of being in the moment, trusting in the goodness of life, and embracing an understanding that things can turn out in any number of ways. Or said a little bit differently, *Choose the world you see, and see the world you choose* (Jonathan Lockwood Huie). And yet another variation, *I'll see it when I believe it.*

---

[1] For more information on the Law of Attraction visit: livinglifefully.com/lawofattraction

[2] Namely, helpguide.org/articles/anxiety/how-to-stop-worrying

SECTION 3: THE SCIENCE BEHIND AGING – AND BEING HAPPY ABOUT IT

Chapter 18: What Does Science Say About Living Longer Than We Think We Will?

An eye-popping statistic from the medical journal, Lancet, has predicted that many 50-year-olds living in Great Britain are only halfway through their lives. In a recent book, *When We're 64: Your Guide to a Greater Later Life,* Louise Ansari, Director of Communications at the United Kingdom's Center for Ageing Better, cites this statistic and others when writing that getting older does not have to mean it all goes downhill. She cautions that most of us are not ready for these extra years.

She documents strategies and tips in her book for us to prepare for the strong likelihood we will live longer than we anticipate, at least from a British point-of-view. Preparation, anticipation, and prevention appear to be the three themes resonating in her recommendations.

I thought it would be helpful to describe her tips for transforming our later years for us to be better prepared for the inevitable changes that occur in our aging bodies. Although they come from a researcher and "anti-aging" expert in Great Britain, we can assume these recommendations have universal appeal:

- Reversing muscle mass loss through physical activity and simple exercises – 30 minutes of moderate aerobic exercise a day. Whether it is sports, shopping and carrying the groceries home, heavy gardening, walking up a flight of stairs 20 times a day, or even standing on one foot when brushing your teeth.

- Keep it easy to get around – the author touts the "20-minute rule" – where can you reach within 20 minutes of walking, driving, public transportation, or bicycling – and prepare yourself for what can happen when you no longer want or are able to drive by making necessary modifications in your home in advance (a walk-in shower, cupboards within easy reach).

- Mental stimulation and improvements in cognitive health – take up a new skill or hobby, learn a new language and practice this new skill up to five hours a week – and make sure it is something fun.

- Stay connected to others – whether through clubs or exercise groups – the recommendation is to stay sociable while also being mindful to replenish your circle of friendships, since others may leave. An added suggestion is to keep your network comprised of people of different ages – who offer different perspectives and bring new learning opportunities. And be sure to maintain that healthy relationship with a partner, sharing both common and independent interests while spicing up your sex life along the way.

- Lose extra weight – to reduce the risk of heart disease, stroke, some cancers, and diabetes, learn how to watch caloric intake, with a more current recommendation of 1,600 total calories a day, down from the usual 2,000 for women and 2,500 for men. And, of course, have alcohol in moderation, with some medical professionals now recommending at least two alcohol-free days a week.

- Financial security – the author stresses the importance of being prepared for living longer and making sure our financial resources and savings are enough for us to live comfortably for the extra 10-15 years that come with our cohort generation.

- Be aware of our own *internalized ageism* – a distaste or revulsion about old age. The author references a study at Yale University that showed negative attitudes toward aging – our own and others' – can take seven years off our life. We must resist the stereotypes and negative thinking about getting older. When we lower our expectations and impose false limitations on our functioning, we also limit our ability to manage setbacks and overcome obstacles. Positive thinking about getting older can effectively help us live longer.

Chapter 19: How Can I Better Understand Meaning and Purpose In Life?

A man began running at the age of 90 for the first time. In 2008, he entered his first national running competition and subsequently set 20 world records for older runners, including American and world records in the 90-94 and the 95-99 age ranges. His name was Orville Roberts. He died at age 101 and lived a remarkable 100+ years. His background includes serving as a fighter pilot in WW II and the Korean War, and then a 31-year career as a commercial airline pilot.

This gentleman survived bypass surgery and at the age of 93, he had a stroke that left him paralyzed on his left side. He did not give up running, though, and instead underwent the most intense rehabilitation he could persuade his physician to provide. Within months he returned to running. His philosophy was *Never, never give up.*

Another inspirational person is Julia Hawkins, lovingly called "Hurricane" by her friends. Julia is also a record holder; she holds the world record for the fastest 100-meter dash in the 100-104 age group, which she won at the Track and Field National Masters Championships in 2017. And, like Orville Roberts, she also started running late – at age 100. She was a competitive biker until there were no other women whom she could compete against and so she turned to sprinting. She overcame fears of embarrassing herself and her family, even of dying from the intense physical activity. She even once said she would make plans in case she *didn't come back* after a race. But, she faced her challenges and her adversity and said, *I looked that fear in the face and I ran.*

A third person who displayed a fantastic accomplishment is Roderick Sewell. He is the first double amputee to complete the Ironman Triathlon World Championship. That's a 2.4-mile swim, a 112-mile bike race (he kneeled on a handcycle), and a 26-mile marathon (using prostheses and running blades). Because he was born without tibias (the large bone in our calves) he had both legs amputated above the knee before his second birthday. On top of this, at just age eight he and his mother were homeless. Yet, he became involved with the Challenged Athletes Foundation and now manages his own fitness studio to train athletes.

Who knows what motivates these people or countless other individuals – many are in their 70's, 80's, and 90's and they get up every day to push themselves off the couch and take on new, daring adventures and physical demands. One likely possibility is the desire to stay connected to others, to stay committed to activity that provides meaning and purpose, and to be able to wake up each morning and ask themselves, *What is my goal for today – what do I want to accomplish?*

We need to remember the lesson on longevity we have learned from centenarians: hold on to – or find – whatever it is that offers a sense of meaning and purpose in life.

Chapter 20: Age Is Only a Number

Now, this is an unusual story about Emile Ratelband. When the story came out a few years ago, he was a single man from Holland working in television. He was unhappy at 69 – he could not get dates from online sites because when prospects found out about his age, they lost interest.

He felt age discrimination – his age affected his ability to work, to get a bank loan for a new house, and find dates. So, he petitioned to the Dutch court to legally change his age – to 49. He argued that at a time when people can change their names or even their gender, opting for a different age should be allowed. *When I'm 69, I am limited. If I'm 49, then I can buy a new house, drive a different car, I can take up more work*, he told the British Broadcasting Service.

But the Dutch court disagreed, saying, Mr. Ratelband is at liberty to *feel* 20 years younger and he can certainly act according to his desired age, but amending his date of birth would cause 20 years of his records to vanish from the Dutch register.

Of course, we cannot change our age and we should not lie about it, but the key point about this story is that we can *feel* younger than our age. Our chronological age, based on the passage of time, is certainly different from our biological or health age. Chronological age is actually a poor predictor of survival and, ironically, its predictive value goes down the closer we approach centenarian status. Biological age, on the other hand, is defined as a measure of how the biological aging process has impacted our body and can be defined by what researchers call *frailty indices* – measures of how well different parts of our body work, such as lung capacity or short term memory – and it is actually a better predictor of survival or mortality. The best part is, although we cannot change how many times the Earth has travelled around the sun since our birth (that is, our chronological age), we *can* impact our biological age with the health-related decisions we make[1].

Regardless of our age, let's remember our senior years can be the best times of our lives. We have the maturity, wisdom, and independence to stay positive about these years. We can always create a mental picture of someone younger than our actual age, just like Emile Ratelband, even if we cannot officially change it.

Most importantly, we want to take control of our future and commit to moving forward, no matter how many bumps we encounter along the way. With losses of loved ones, we move forward. With a secure retirement and good health and with bodies that do not cooperate, we still look forward. Our beauty and worth are in our essence, attitude, and our outlook. And, as noted in an earlier chapter, the best part is no one can take this attitude away from us. It is ours to keep – forever.

---

[1] Jarreau, P. (2019). *How Old Are You, Really? Meet Your Biological Age*. Lifeapps. lifeapps.io/brain/how-old-are-you-really-meet-your-biological-age

BIOGRAPHY

Joseph M. Casciani, PhD, is the founder and Chief Curator of the **Living to 100 Club** (livingto100.club), the author's new voice for delivering insights and inspiration about aging with a positive mindset – no matter how hard the journey. The desire to share these insights and this outlook on aging does not come from seminars or a few years in the field. They are the culmination of the author's experience with older adults and their families, the paid and unpaid caregivers of older adults, writing and public speaking, and the hundreds of mental health professionals and scores of hospitals and long-term care facilities with whom he has worked with since the early 1980s.

He has an almost 40-year career in the field of clinical geropsychology. He attended San Diego State University for his Master's degree and U.S. International University (now Alliant) for his doctorate. He was awarded the first contract from the California Department of Aging in 1982 to develop training manuals and curricula for the state's long-term care facilities on aging and mental health topics. Subsequently, he became the co-founder and president of a multi-state mental health group, providing services in LTC settings. For 16 years he was responsible for program development and the delivery of clinical services to patients in over 800 nursing facilities, in eight states, along with operating practice management organizations in several states, developing clinical programs and protocols for mental health services in long-term care settings, and sponsoring online training programs and webinars in the field of aging for health care professionals.

He began his own group practices, Concept Healthcare and CoHealth Psychology Services, in 2007 to provide training for those working with older adults. Soon afterward, his companies managed and supported practitioners delivering mental health services in LTC facilities, in two states. After 12 years, he transferred ownership of his professional corporations to a new company in 2019. He is now semi-retired with a hand in supporting the new owner and keeping a strategic focus on the Living to 100 Club while writing, public speaking, and consulting.

Dr. Casciani is the co-editor of *Geropsychology and Long Term Care: A Practitioner's Guide* (Springer, 2008), and author of *The Handbook of Health and Behavior* (Concept Healthcare, 2012). He is a former Board member of the *Council of Professional Geropsychology Training Programs* and is a past President of *Psychologists in Long Term Care*. Dr. Casciani has presented at several professional association meetings, including the American Society on Aging, American Medical Directors Association, and the American Psychological Association on a range of topics in aging and mental health.

The founder of the **Living to 100 Club** resides in San Diego, California, USA, and can be reached at Info@Livingto100.Club.

RECOMMENDED BOOKS AND RESOURCES

Books

1. *The 36-Hour Day: A Family Guide to Caring for People with Dementia and Memory Loss* – Nancy L. Mace

2. *The Blue Zones: 9 Lessons for Living Longer* – Dan Buettner

3. *The Blue Zones Solution* – Dan Buettner

4. *The Cancer Nutrition Center Handbook* – Carolyn Katzin

5. *Caring for Your Parents: AARP Guide* – Hugh Delehanty

6. *How to Break the Habit of Being Yourself* – Dr. Joe Dispenza

7. *Living to Be 100* – Michael Howard

8. *The Longevity Paradox: How to Die Young at a Ripe Old Age (The Plant Paradox)* – Steve Gundry

9. *Love for Imperfect Things* – Haemin Sunim

10. *Raising Your Aging Parent* – Kenneth Druck

11. *Restorying Our Lives: Personal Growth Through Autobiographical Reflection* – Gary Kenyon

12. *When We're 64: Your Guide to a Greater, Later Life* – Louise Ansari

13. *What Retirees Want* – Ken Dychtwald

Articles

14. Barnosky, A. R., Hoddy, K. K., Unterman, T. G. & Varady, K. A. (2014). Intermittent fasting vs daily calorie restriction for type 2 diabetes prevention: a review of human findings. *Translational Research*, 164(4), 302-311.

15. Goodrick, C. L., Ingram, D. K., Reynolds, M. A., Freeman, J. R. & Cider, N. L. (1982). Effects of Intermittent Feeding Upon Growth and Life Span in Rats. *Gerontology*, 28, 233-241.

16. Heilbronn, L.K., Smith, S.R., Martin, C.K., Anton, S.D. & Ravussin, E. (2005). Alternate-day fasting in nonobese subjects: effects on body weight, body composition, and energy metabolism. *Am J Clin Nutr.* 81(1), 69-73.

17. Ho, K. Y., Veldhuis, J. D., Johnson, M. L., Furlanetto, R., Evans, W. S., Alberti, K. G. & Thorner, M. O. (1988). Fasting enhances growth hormone secretion and amplifies the complex rhythms of growth hormone secretion in man. *The Journal of clinical investigation*, 81(4), 968-975.

18. Johnson, J. B., Summer, W., Cutler, R. G., Martin, B., Hyun, D. H., Dixit, V. D., Pearson, M., Nassar, M., Telljohann, R., Maudsley, S., Carlson, O., John, S., Laub, D. R. & Mattson, M. P. (2007). Alternate day calorie restriction improves clinical findings and reduces markers of oxidative stress and inflammation in overweight adults with moderate asthma. *Free radical biology & medicine*, 42(5), 665-674.

19. Lee, J., Duan, W., Long, J. M., Ingram, D. K. & Mattson, M. P. (2000). Dietary restriction increases the number of newly generated neural cells, and induces BDNF expression, in the dentate gyrus of rats. *Journal of molecular neuroscience*, 15(2), 99-108.

20. Martin, B., Mattson, M. P. & Maudsley, S. (2006). Caloric restriction and intermittent fasting: two potential diets for successful brain aging. *Ageing research reviews*, 5(3), 332-353.

21. Martin, B., Pearson, M., Brenneman, R., Golden, E., Wood, W., Prabhu, V., Becker, K. G., Mattson, M. P., & Maudsley, S. (2009). Gonadal transcriptome alterations in response to dietary energy intake: sensing the reproductive environment. *PloS one*, 4(1).

22. Reis de Azevedo, F., Ikeoka, D. & Caramelli, B. (2013). Effects of intermittent fasting on metabolism in men. *Revista da Associação Médica Brasileira*, 59(2), 167-173.

23. Varady, K. A., Bhutani, S., Church, E. C. & Klempel, M. C. (2009). Short-term modified alternate-day fasting: a novel dietary strategy for weight loss and cardioprotection in obese adults. *The American journal of clinical nutrition*, 90(5), 1138-1143.

Websites

24. Gunners, K. (2017). *How Intermittent Fasting Can Help You Lose Weight*. Heathline. www.healthline.com/nutrition/intermittent-fasting-and-weight-loss

25. Harvard Chan School. (2017). *In Pursuit of Healthy Aging*. The Harvard Gazette. news.harvard.edu/gazette/story/2017/11/intermittent-fasting-may-be-center-of-increasing-lifespan

26. Jarreau, P. (2019). *How Old Are You, Really? Meet Your Biological Age*. Lifeapps. lifeapps.io/brain/how-old-are-you-really-meet-your-biological-age

27. Mayo clinic staff. (2020). *Caregiver stress: Tips for taking care of yourself*. Mayoclinic. www.mayoclinic.org/healthy-lifestyle/stress-management/in-depth/caregiver-stress/art-20044784

28. National Institute on Aging. (2017). *Sexuality in Later Life*. nia.nih.gov/health/sexuality-later-life

29. Public Health Agency of Canada. (September 2006). *Seniors and Aging - Sexual Activity*. publications.gc.ca/collections/collection_2007/hc-sc/H13-7-15-2006E.pdf

30. Roan, S. (2010). *Life span may be as wide as your smile*. Los Angeles Times. latimes.com/archives/la-xpm-2010-mar-29-la-he-capsule-20100329-story

31. Segal, M. & Smith, M. (2019). *Better Sex as You Age.* HelpGuide. helpguide.org/articles/alzheimers-dementia-aging/better-sex-as-you-age.htm

Other resources

Lives Well Lived – DVD, produced by Sky Bergman

Memory Loss Fidget & Therapy Pillow from Amazon

Made in the USA
Monee, IL
18 June 2020